The Layman's Guide to a Healthier You

A simple step by step guide to change your life and improve your health

Lisa Kafer

Lisa Kafer
Clean Food, Clean You
PO Box 794
Carthage, MO 64836

Cleanfoodcleanyou@gmail.com
www.cleanfoodcleanyou.com
www.facebook.com/417cleanfoodcleanyou

ISBN 9781795211376

DEDICATION

This book is dedicated to my dear friends Dave Gore and Jeanne Achey, who I lost too soon to the ravages of cancer. I miss them both. If I'd known then what I know now, perhaps I could have done more to help. It is also dedicated to all those who have lost loved ones to cancer and other preventable diseases. My mission is to help teach the world there's a better path to health for life, and my prayer is that *The Layman's Guide to a Healthier You* will touch lives and be of value to many.

CONTENTS

ACKNOWLEDGMENTS

I would like to acknowledge the many pioneers in modern medicine who stepped out of their comfort zones to pursue true health by learning, and then teaching what Hippocrates knew decades ago before modern medicine decided to treat symptoms with drugs. I learned so much from amazing health practitioners like Dr. David Brownstein, Dr. Tom O'Bryan, Dr. Gabriel Cousens, Dr. Russell Blaylock, Dr. Mariza Snyder and many others. I only hope to touch as many lives as them and play a small part in changing the face of healthcare to a more holistic, more food-based natural system.

INTRODUCTION

Are you ready to enjoy a vibrant healthy life? Are you overwhelmed with all the information on health and wellness and don't know where to start? Have you been bombarded with books and articles on this subject? I know I have, and this is why I have put together all the great information I've learned in *The Layman's Guide to a Healthier You*--a comprehensive, easy to implement guide.

In this book, I'm going to show you how to look great and feel better! I'm going to show you how to eat healthy for life without giving up your family favorites. I'm going to teach you how to eat healthy with a busy schedule; because to be truly healthy and vibrant, you have to eat healthy more than once in a while. It has to be a lifestyle change.

I'm going to teach you some natural health solutions for you and your family. Besides teaching you what to eat, I'll share some recipes to get you started. I'll also teach you what ingredients and chemicals to avoid in your foods, cosmetics, personal hygiene, and cleaning products to have a healthier environment and a healthier body. And I'm going to show you how to reset your body for more vibrant living and weight loss.

As a Healthy Lifestyle Coach and cooking instructor and a student of healthy living, I have read and tested hundreds of the best books, blogs, articles and webinars about living a healthy lifestyle. Busy moms and dads, students, and many others who struggle with living a healthy lifestyle in our toxic world have already experienced great success by implementing the tips and tricks found in this helpful how-to guide. Thousands have improved their health, energy, and sleep, and have shed those unwanted pounds using the tips I share.

My genetics has provided me the great fortune to have lived most of my life tall and thin. But, at the age of 40, I found myself in a new relationship and my husband and I wanted to have a child together. Just shy of my 44th birthday, I gave birth to my second child. My first daughter was about to celebrate her 17th birthday. I sailed through the pregnancy and delivered a beautiful baby girl, all naturally. It was several years after that I was feeling badly about my body. For the first time in my life, I was overweight, having to buy larger and larger clothes sizes. I thought I was eating healthy, but I couldn't lose the weight. As I stood in front of the mirror as I got ready for my day, I hated the image staring back at me. I told myself it was just because I was older, and I would never get back into my size 5 jeans. It's just harder to lose weight as you get older. Isn't that what they say? So, I gave away all the size 5 jeans I thought I'd never wear again and tried to reconcile myself to a life in bigger jeans.

Then one day, I was introduced to a 30-day detox program and some education on healthy eating. I decided to give it a try. Over the course of a year, I detoxed twice and ended up losing 35 pounds. I still remember the day I was able to try on a pair of size 5 jeans and they actually fit! I felt amazing! I was sleeping better and had more energy, too. Now, seven years later, at the age of 60, I am still wearing my size 5 jeans. I ride horses, I dance almost every week, I can still do a cartwheel and I feel amazing! It was this journey that showed me my passion in life; to help others achieve their best health ever! It can be done at any age!

I promise that if you follow the how-to guide below, you will experience better overall health for yourself and your family, more energy and weight loss. You will live in a cleaner environment and reduce your toxic load.

You and your kids will be sick less often. You'll spend less time at doctors' appointments and your kids will miss less school. The benefits this book can bring you are too numerous to mention but span the gamut of saving time, money and most important of all giving you a healthier lifestyle. If you have your health, you have everything!

Don't be the person who misses out on opportunities in life because you don't have the energy or you're at home sick or your kids are sick. Be the kind of person other people marvel at. Be the kind of person other people see and say, 'You look amazing! What are you doing?' Be the kind of person who takes action immediately to turn your life around!

The health and wellness tips and tricks you're about to read have been proven to create positive, long-lasting results. All you have to do to take control of your health is to keep reading. I will walk you through it. Each chapter will give you new insight as you strive to live a more vibrant life. Take control of your life right now, make it productive, and enjoy the new life you're creating.

Section 1

Detoxing

Chapter 1

What is Detoxing?

The first step to a healthier you is to rid your body of the heavy metals, chemicals, and environmental toxins we all accumulate in our bodies and to rid our bodies of cravings that make us eat foods we know we shouldn't. When our parents and grandparents were young, detoxing wasn't a thing. But there weren't as many toxins in the world. People ate at home more and cooked with fresh ingredients. These days, due to the many sources of toxins we encounter daily, we all need to detox at least once or twice a year. This doesn't have to be a horrible, starving fast or mean spending hours in the bathroom. Depending on the level of your toxic load, it can be a very easy, pain-free experience. Worst case, you might experience a bit of constipation or a headache.

We encounter toxins in the foods we eat, in the form of genetically modified soy, corn and sugar beet sugar that are used in just about every boxed and processed food on the market, through the increase in the amount of pesticides and herbicides sprayed on our crops, the antibiotics and hormones in the animal products we consume and the drugs and other toxins that leach into our soil. Then there are the chemicals made into "food products" or put into food that aren't even real food and weren't meant for human consumption.

We are also exposed to hundreds of chemicals a day from the hygiene and cosmetic products we use on our bodies and the cleaning products in our homes, along with fragranced candles and room fresheners, plastics and carpet. Another source of toxins is the electromagnetic energy we are bombarded with daily from the electronics that dominate our lives: computers, cell phones, Wi-Fi, microwaves and cell towers. Newborn babies born today have been tested for chemical toxins and it was found that babies are born with over 230 toxic chemicals in their bodies. These toxins come from the toxins in the parents, including the food eaten by the mother and from environmental toxins. Whatever the mother consumes or uses on her body is absorbed by the baby. This may be one of the reasons that childhood cancers are on the rise. So, regardless of whether you are sick or well, heavy or thin, everyone should detox. It is the best place to start to live a healthy life.

You might be asking what exactly is a detox and what does it do? How does it work? In short, detoxing is a reset for your body, primarily your gut flora, your fat cells, and your major organs. Let me explain. There are basically 9 things a detox does for you.

1. Detoxing heals the gut and gives your digestive tract a rest because, during a detox, you are eating foods that are easily digested. About 65% of your metabolism is used to digest food. That's one reason you might feel like you need a nap after eating a big meal. Your body spends a lot of energy digesting food. With constant over-eating or eating hard to digest foods, your body never gets a rest. With the hybridized wheat that we eat in the form of bread, pasta, and processed foods, more and more people are being diagnosed with leaky gut, which has been shown to cause gut issues like Crohn's disease, IBS (irritable bowel syndrome) and celiac

disease and can also lead to autoimmune diseases like RA (Rheumatoid Arthritis), MS and others.

2. Giving the gut a rest and strengthening the gut flora by detoxing can help the gut heal. Detoxing balances blood sugar. By controlling the amount of sugar--and carbs that turn into sugar--and thereby eliminating spikes in blood sugar, the stress on your liver and pancreas is reduced. In our discussion about blood sugar I mention the glycemic index of different foods. Glycemic Index is a system that ranks foods on a scale from 1 to 100 based on the carbohydrates in the food and their effect on blood-sugar (blood glucose) levels.

3. Detoxing balances pH and reduces inflammation. Balancing pH is critical to staying healthy. A higher pH (more acidic) is a breeding ground for cancer cells and inflammation. Chronic inflammation is the basis for just about all disease, including heart disease, arthritis, muscle, and joint issues and many other diseases. A more alkaline environment is much healthier for your cells; reduced inflammation goes a long way to healing the body.

4. Detoxing can lower cholesterol. Even though it has been proven that chronic inflammation and not high cholesterol is the leading cause of heart disease, changing your diet and ridding your body of toxins does tend to lower the bad cholesterol in most people.

5. Detoxing strengthens the immune system. You may know that 70% to 80% of your immune system is in your gut. When you improve your gut flora, the number of healthy gut bacteria increases; you are strengthening your immune system. Since I started detoxing and eating clean, I have not been sick at all.

6. Detoxing helps reduce the stress on the detoxing organs in the body--the liver and kidneys. We put such a heavy burden on our bodies when we consume things like caffeine, alcohol, sugar GMO's and processed food, that our liver and kidneys can be overburdened. Besides giving our digestive tract a rest, we are also cleansing our liver and kidneys and giving them a rest. This will help eliminate fatty liver disease and other issues.

7. Another important aspect of a detox is to improve your gut flora. In other words, you want to increase the good bacteria and decrease the bad bacteria in your gut, so your food is properly digested, and nutrients are absorbed. Undigested food causes intestinal toxemia, which occurs when large particles of undigested food enter the small intestine and colon.

Since these parts of the digestive tract were not meant to handle large quantities of undigested food, the partially digested food mass becomes a fertile breeding ground for bad bacteria and yeast fermentation. Each nutrient degrades in its own unique way. Proteins putrefy, carbohydrates ferment, and fats become rancid due to the workings of intestinal bacteria. These bacteria then produce harmful by-products that damage the intestines, reduce nutrient absorption, create excess gas and bloating, and lead to persistent diarrhea.

On top of that, mild to intense stomach pains (the result of muscle cramping and excessive gas) accompany this process. Prolonged intestinal toxemia may be a major contributing factor in the onset of irritable bowel syndrome and Crohn's disease.

8. Probably the most obvious benefit of detoxing is that it reduces toxic load, which helps us lose weight. We have already mentioned the high number of toxins we take in through our skin, through breathing, and through eating.

   Detoxing helps rid the body of these toxins, which are stored in our fat cells; typically, the visceral fat cells in the belly. This is why people tend to lose weight when they do a detox. When the toxic load is reduced, the fat cells have no purpose.

   This is also why you may reach a plateau in your weight loss program. This is why you can't eat badly and just exercise it away. The fat cells are doing their job by holding on to the toxins to protect the major organs. Until you rid your body of the toxins, you will not lose that visceral fat.

9. The last thing a detox can do for you is to reduce the cravings that make you eat what you know you shouldn't eat--like cravings for sugar and carbs. Sugar is more addictive than cocaine and it makes our body very acidic. A good detox can reduce those cravings, which goes a long way towards helping us get healthy.

As you can see, detoxing has many benefits for the body and affects all areas of the body, from cells to muscles, digestion, brain, and organs. It is vital for everyone, no matter how well you think you may eat.

Just by virtue of living in this modern world of ours, we all take in many chemical and electromagnetic toxins as well as heavy metals. There are many different types of detoxes out there, but I recommend a 30-day full body detox. In the next chapter, we'll discuss what is involved in a detox and what foods to avoid when doing a detox to get you the best results.

Chapter 2

How Do I Detox?

So, what does it look like to do a detox? From my research on this subject, I have determined that the best detox is a 30-day process. It involves drinking a meal-replacement shake for 2 meals a day and eating a clean meal for the third, with healthy snacks, if needed, in between. This schedule gives your digestive system that much-needed rest I was talking about.

A good plant-based (non-soy) protein shake with lots of vitamins and minerals is a good choice. I also recommend milk thistle or dandelion tea to help cleanse the liver and kidneys. Prebiotics and probiotics are also extremely important because these contain digestive enzymes and the good bacteria your gut needs to properly digest your food and to help with maximum absorption of nutrients. I have found that many pre- and probiotics do not contain strong enough enzymes to survive the stomach acid. So, I recommend one that can make it to the colon, as this is where they are most needed.

What to Avoid When Detoxing

A full-blown detox would ideally include avoiding chemicals in personal hygiene and cosmetic products, and in cleaning products, but this will be covered in another chapter. Here we will discuss foods and drinks to avoid when detoxing.

Most of the things I'm going to mention here should ideally be avoided altogether. They do damage to your body and serve no beneficial purpose. Having said that, if you can give them up for 30-days, you may find you never want to go back to them again. If there are some you still want to consume, I would recommend introducing one at a time back into your diet and see how they make you feel. Once your body gets used to NOT having to deal with them, you may notice a more severe reaction to them. I'll explain more as we discuss each of these foods.

The things most important to eliminate, especially during a detox, are:

1. Gluten

2. GMO's (Soy, corn and sugar beet sugar are the three biggies)

3. Sugar

4. Dairy

5. Caffeine & Alcohol

6. MSG, Nitrates & Artificial Sweeteners,

7. Bad Fats

8. Peanuts and Peanut Butter

9. High Glycemic Fruits

10. Vinegar and Products that contain Vinegar, (except Organic Apple Cider Vinegar)

11. White Potatoes

12. Farm-raised Fish and Seafood

13. Commercially grown Beef and Chicken – eat only Grass-Fed and Free-Range

14. All Pork and Pork Products

This may seem like a daunting list and you may be asking, "What is left to eat"? In the next few chapters, I will explain why you want to avoid each of these above-mentioned items and what you can eat instead. I promise you won't feel deprived or starving.

If you follow a good 30-day detox as I've mentioned, you will see some amazing results. I've seen diabetics lower their blood-sugar enough to have to reduce or eliminate their insulin. Just about everyone I've seen participate in this type of detox loses weight.

I lost over 35 pounds, myself. There have been some who couldn't walk down a flight of stairs who—through detoxing--experienced relief from joint pain. Most people find they sleep better, wake more refreshed, have better brain function, get rid of bloating and gas and have more energy.

Because this is a whole-body cleanse, it really does restart your body systems and starts you on a wellness journey. It's important to do this detox with support – with a friend or loved one who shares your goals. You can keep each other accountable and help each other through any difficult days when you're tempted to cheat. I offer a comprehensive detox program complete with coaching, meal ideas, recipes, and education. Find out more on my website at:

www.cleanfoodcleanyou.com

In the next chapter, I'll dig deep into the "bad" foods and explain why they are bad. Then we'll cover the good foods that will nourish your body.

Section 2

Let Food be thy Medicine

Chapter 3

The Bad Foods and Why They are Bad

GLUTEN

As you probably know, gluten is a family of proteins found in rye, barley, and wheat. They are thick and gooey and make things stick together when baked. Wheat is the most commonly consumed gluten-forming grain. Wheat has been hybridized to the point that it is extremely difficult for just about anyone to digest.

Over the past 50 years, wheat strains have been altered to make the wheat resistant to environmental stresses such as drought. Gone are the fields of tall wheat we used to refer to as amber waves of grain. Much of the current wheat supply, about 99% of it, is a hybridized dwarf variety that produces a higher quantity of the gluten genes that today are associated with celiac disease and other gut issues. There are also recent studies that show that leaky gut causes autoimmune diseases and gluten has been closely linked with leaky gut.

The trickiest part of avoiding gluten altogether is in finding it in foods you wouldn't think would have gluten in them. Food products like salad dressings, seasonings, season mixes, and sauces may contain gluten, along with condiments and many other food products.

The best way to totally avoid gluten is to steer clear of processed food completely. If you can tolerate a little gluten, you probably don't have to worry about the little bit in salad dressings and such, but I would recommend avoiding any wheat, barley and rye products including breads and pastas. There are many great alternatives out there.

If you feel you can't do without your bread, choose a whole sprouted grain, wheat-free bread. For making pancakes and waffles, you can buy gluten-free all-purpose flour. Making your own risen baked goods is a bit trickier and will require a good recipe that has been tested. But gluten-free bakers are becoming more prevalent and it is easier to find good gluten-free baked goods than in years past.

Check with your local health food store. They will most likely carry locally made gluten-free items. If you choose to make your own, there are lots of alternative flours made from gluten-free grains and beans like oats, brown rice, coconut, garbanzo beans, amaranth, cassava, and others. There are also flours made from nuts like almonds.

There are two other very important reasons to avoid wheat products.

1. Wheat, although non-GMO, is typically sprayed with glyphosate herbicide right before harvesting. Spraying with glyphosate kills the wheat plant which makes harvesting the wheat grains much easier. So, besides containing more gluten, the wheat is covered in a toxic chemical herbicide.

2. Most commercial products made from wheat contain a carcinogenic compound called bromine. Years ago, bakeries put iodine in bread as an anti-caking agent. Iodine is an essential nutrient used in every cell in our

bodies. But since the mid-'70s, the cheaper toxic chemical called bromine has been used, instead.

Most of the wheat flour made, which translates to most of the bread and pasta products out there, contains bromine. Bromine and bromide can also be found in some prescription medications, fire retardants used in children's sleepwear and drinks like Mountain Dew and some Gatorade, in the form of brominated vegetable oil. Bromine is also used to kill termites and is an ingredient in swimming pool chemicals.

Bromine is in the chemical family of halides, of which iodine is also a member. Bromine and iodine appear the same to our body, so the iodine receptors in our body will attract the bromine. But, as I mentioned, bromine is a carcinogenic compound and the body has no known use for it. If a person is iodine-deficient, which studies show most people are, the body will replace the iodine deficit with bromine. Bromine promotes the formation of goiter, but iodine prevents goiter and has anti-carcinogenic properties.

Webster's dictionary defines bromine as "a nonmetallic halogen element that is isolated as a deep red corrosive toxic volatile liquid of disagreeable odor". Besides the gut-damaging gluten in our wheat products, we are also ingesting a known carcinogen.

To detox properly, you should eliminate gluten (and bromine) from your diet for 30 days. After that, reintroduce a few bromine-free gluten products, if you must. But be aware of what they do to your body and how you feel after you eat them. Most likely, you will not feel good. It's possible that you won't feel the effects for hours or days. If you can eliminate gluten from your diet completely, your body will thank you for it.

GMO's – Genetically Modified Organisms

According to the USDA, there are now more than 40 crops considered to be or are being monitored as "high risk" GMO crops and 4 crops that -- you can pretty much guarantee -- have been genetically modified. These four crops are corn, soy, sugar beets, and cotton. So, what exactly does that mean? That means that these crops have been modified to produce their own pesticides and to be resistant to glyphosate, the key ingredient in Roundup herbicides.

What does that mean to us? It means that farmers who grow GMO crops can spray their crops with higher doses of toxic herbicides to kill the weeds that are becoming more and more resistant to Roundup.

That means your corn, soy and sugar beets and all products made with these crops, have absorbed this toxic chemical. It can't be washed off. It's not ON the food, it's IN the food. And if the bugs won't eat it, why should we? Something else to consider is that more than just GMO crops are being sprayed with Roundup. And as we've already mentioned, wheat is a crop that is frequently sprayed right before harvest.

To make matters worse, because the weeds are becoming resistant to Roundup and have become "super weeds", Monsanto, who makes Roundup and controls all the GMO seeds, has come up with a stronger version of Roundup containing the chemical 2,4-D an ingredient found in Agent

Orange. Most baby boomers will remember that Agent Orange was used in Vietnam in herbicidal warfare.

Glyphosate has been associated with endocrine disruption. The endocrine system refers to the collection of glands that secrete our hormones, so this means glyphosate disrupts the hormones. It has also been associated with reproductive issues, neurotoxicity, cancer, and DNA damage.

Recent studies have shown that couples who couldn't conceive a child, eliminated GMO food products from their diets and were then able to conceive. Do you want your kids ingesting this toxin? Seventy percent of foods sold in the supermarket contain genetically modified ingredients.

Over 5 million children in the US are suffering from food allergies; a problem that can be tied to the development of GMO processed foods for infants and children. According to Dr. Deanna Osborn, DO, in her book *Dr. Deanna's Healing Handbook*, "Most baby formula is made from cow's milk, and the great majority of milk-based formulas are produced from milk taken from cows injected with bovine growth hormone, with GMO corn sweeteners added. If the baby is allergic to milk-based formula, the four, bestselling soy-based formulas are made from GMO soy. The (WIC) program provides formula to over 2 million newborns in the United States. The WIC program ONLY provides formulas that contain genetically engineered soy or rBGH derived milk."

Even organically grown soybeans naturally contain "anti-nutrients" that keep the body from absorbing nutrients from our food. Traditional fermentation destroys these anti-nutrients, which allows your body to enjoy soy's nutritional benefits. However, most Westerners do not consume fermented soy. Most consume soy in the form of soymilk, tofu, TVP (Textured Vegetable Protein), and soy infant formula, none of which are fermented.

Soy's anti-nutrients are quite potent. One of the biggest anti-nutrients is a phytoestrogen. Drinking just two glasses of soymilk daily provides enough phytoestrogen to alter a woman's menstrual cycle.

But if you feed soy to your infant or child, these effects are magnified a thousand-fold. Infants fed soy formula may have up to 20,000 times more estrogen circulating through their bodies as those fed other formulas.

You should NEVER feed your infant a soy-based formula! In fact, infants fed soy formula take in an estimated five birth control pills' worth of estrogen every day.

There are other issues associated with consuming soy. Among those are vitamin deficiencies, especially vitamins B12 and D and thyroid issues. If you'd like more information about soy, I recommend doing further research. There have been many studies, and lots written on the subject, more than I can cover here. Just know that unfermented soy should be avoided completely, especially by children.

Most people are aware of the dangers to your health of consuming genetically modified high fructose corn syrup. Not only is it made from GMO corn, it is a form of sugar that has to be converted by the liver to be used by the body. Fructose is the type of sugar found in fruit. Smaller amounts of fructose from fruit can be fine because, when you eat fruit you are getting fiber and nutrients along with a small amount of fructose. When you consume soda, candy and any of the tens of thousands of products that contain large doses of fructose, the liver can be overloaded, and the fructose can be converted to fat. In the long term, this fat accumulation can lead to serious health problems, such as fatty liver disease and type 2 diabetes. This is the worst sweetener you can consume.

The big issue with this is that it is found in just about every processed food product. It is found in many things you may not think about. Foods like peanut butter, catsup, salad dressings, drinks of all kinds, breakfast cereal, and the more common things like pop and candy. But there are other forms of GMO sugar you may not be aware of. If a product lists sugar in its ingredients list, unless it specifically states cane sugar or organic cane sugar, it is most likely sugar beet sugar. Beets are a wonderful vegetable full of nutrients. But beets absorb everything – good and bad. Genetically modified sugar beets are grown from seeds injected with viral and/or bacterial genes and the plants are heavily sprayed with Roundup, so they absorb all the toxins in this product. Then they are processed to form white sugar; not only full of toxic chemicals, but also devoid of any of the nutrients found in beets. This sugar should be avoided.

SUGAR

We've already talked about GMO sugar beet sugar and high fructose corn syrup, so we won't cover that again here, but what about refined cane sugar? Unfortunately, this isn't any better for you. Refined sugar has been stripped of all nutrients and drains and leaches the body of precious vitamins and minerals. Sugar eaten every day produces a continuously acidic condition which affects every organ in the body. This acidic environment is exactly where cancer grows best. Cancer feeds on sugar. That is why it is very important to make sure your body is pH balanced and why this is one of the biggest goals of a detox program.

Doctors know that cancer feeds on sugar. When they test a person for cancer, they inject sugar and watch where it goes in the body. If there is cancer, the sugar will gravitate to the cancerous cells. Initially, sugar is stored in the liver. A daily intake of refined sugar makes the liver expand like a balloon. When the liver has reached its capacity, the excess sugar is returned to the blood in the form of fatty acids.

These are stored in the most inactive areas, the belly, the buttocks, and the thighs. In contrast, unrefined sugars contain minerals the body needs. So, you don't have to completely give up sweets. There are alternative sweeteners that we'll talk about in another chapter.

DAIRY

Milk - Does a body good?? RIGHT? Not really!! We've already talked about the rBGH (bovine growth hormone) in most milk. And guess who owns the company that makes bovine growth hormone? Yup! Monsanto.

Besides being very hard to digest, milk causes your body to be acidic and causes inflammation. It is also mucus forming. Let's think about this for a minute. What is milk? Webster Dictionary defines it this way: "A white liquid produced by a woman to feed her baby or by female animals to feed their young". That is, milk is species-specific. That means that as a food, it is designed perfectly for each species' own offspring. Humans are the only species known to drink another mammal's milk.

Cow's milk is designed to help a baby calf grow big and strong very fast, and then they don't drink it anymore. Do we want our kids growing like a calf? Do we really need to drink milk all our lives? We don't. If your dog had puppies, would you drink her milk? Probably not!

But what about calcium, you might ask? Milk makes for strong bones and teeth, right? Did you know you can get more calcium from a cup of broccoli than you can from a glass of milk? We only absorb a small percentage of the calcium found in milk.

Dr. David Brownstein states that, in his experience, he has seen that up to half of all children and more than 80 percent of adults, exhibit antibodies to a protein in milk called casein. A milk allergy can manifest in many ways. The most common symptoms are gastrointestinal problems, including diarrhea, bloating, gassiness and constipation.

However, there are many other symptoms related to dairy: problems including asthma, autism, behavioral issues, headaches, chest pains, dry skin, hives, rashes, stuffy nose, snoring, runny nose, and sneezing. Keep in mind, if you eat dairy and nothing happens right away, this does not mean you are not allergic to milk. Most food allergy reactions may take hours or even days to occur.

Is dairy bad for everyone? Not necessarily. But conventional dairy products, which contain synthetic hormones and antibiotics, should be avoided during a detox and if you can cut out dairy altogether, your body will love you for it, just like cutting out gluten.

ALCOHOL and CAFFEINE

Alcohol and caffeine should be avoided during a detox. Alcohol stresses the liver and the kidneys. Caffeine decreases nutrient absorption, dulls the taste buds and makes the body extremely acidic. And, if you recall, one of the main goals of a detox is to balance your body's pH.

So, ditch the coffee and caffeinated teas for this 30-day period. If you are a heavy coffee drinker or drink a lot of caffeine from another source, this will be the time when you may experience headaches. But hang in there, this phase won't last long.

Alcohol stresses the liver because, when it reaches the liver, it produces a toxic enzyme called acetaldehyde which can damage liver cells and cause permanent scarring, as well as harm to the brain and stomach lining.

In addition, the liver requires water to work properly. Alcohol dehydrates your liver and forces it to find water from other sources in your body, which can dehydrate your body. This is part of the reason why, after a big night of drinking you can wake up with a major headache.

Alcohol causes changes in the function of the kidneys and makes them less able to filter the blood. Alcohol also affects the ability to regulate fluid and electrolytes in the body. When alcohol dehydrates the body, the drying effect can hinder the normal function of cells and organs, including the kidneys. In addition, alcohol can disrupt hormones that affect kidney function.

We only have one liver and two kidneys, and they are our major detoxing organs. In order to allow them to do their jobs as effectively as possible, it is wise to avoid drinking alcohol and caffeine so they can work to rid the body of the other toxins.

ASPARTAME, NITRATES, MSG

Aspartame is an artificial sweetener used in diet drinks and most diet foods. It was developed by GD Searle Pharmaceuticals in 1981, a company purchased by, guess who??? Monsanto, in 1983. Are you starting to see a pattern here?

Of all adverse reactions to food additives reported to the FDA, 75% of them are attributed to Aspartame. Aspartame and MSG act in the body as neurotransmitters and an overabundance destroys neurons by triggering free radicals which kill brain cells.

Researchers have found a correlation between aspartame consumption and migraine headaches, fatigue, depression, anxiety, and memory loss. Aspartame should be avoided considering the huge spike in neurological diseases like MS, Alzheimer's, brain cancer, Parkinson's and dementia.

Nitrates - Processed meats like ham, hot dogs, bacon and most lunch meat contain many chemicals like nitrates or nitrites, hormones, and antibiotics. Nitrates are also found in many vegetables, so it is a naturally occurring element. So, nitrates in and of themselves are not bad in small quantities but when they are heated to high temperatures and are combined with protein, nitrosamine is produced, which is one of the more potent carcinogens. It has been strongly linked to cancers in the digestive tract, especially colon cancer. Nitrates are just one of the reasons to avoid processed meats. Many are made from all sorts of animal parts that serve no other function and are full of chemicals you want to avoid.

TOXIC OILS – Bad Fats

What do I mean by toxic oils, you might ask? The food industry has really pulled one over on us when it comes to oils. For years they have told us that margarine is better for us than butter. Margarine is one molecule shy of being plastic. They have told us that hydrogenated anything is better for our hearts: canola oil, safflower oil, corn oil, peanut oil – they sell it by the gallon! These, we are told, are "heart healthy".

If truth be told, these oils contribute immensely to heart disease because they cause inflammation, which is the leading cause of heart disease and just about every other disease. That's why fried foods are so bad for you. It's not the fact that the food is fried as much as it is the oil used in the frying process.

The oils I recommend are avocado oil, flaxseed oil, extra virgin olive oil--if you can find it pure--and coconut oil. More about coconut oil later. It is simply amazing stuff! Be aware that you will want to avoid not only these bad fats but food products that contain them or are cooked in them. Processed foods and food products contain these toxic ingredients. Fried food is a no-no unless you cook it yourself in one of the healthy oils. Read your labels.

PEANUTS and PEANUT BUTTER

Many people have an allergy to peanuts. They are not actually allergic to the peanut itself, but the toxic fungus found within the peanut. Peanuts are one of eight major food allergens in the U.S. The peanut allergy can usually be linked to the natural mold aflatoxin, which can damage the liver. This aflatoxin forms because peanuts grow under the ground. Aflatoxin is a potent carcinogen. Removing this so-called healthy food from your diet also means you are cutting down on the toxic load exposure from the environment.

Other than aflatoxin, there are even more toxins associated with peanuts. Non-organic peanuts and peanut butter are also contaminated with pesticides. This is a concern because peanuts have a very light shell, which pesticides can easily permeate. Conventional peanuts have a very high pesticide rate, as well as other chemical contaminants.

Yet another issue with peanuts is that 30% of the fatty acids in peanut butter are the Omega-6 fatty acid, linoleic acid. Omega-6 fatty acids in the diet are associated with inflammation and an increased risk of cardiovascular disease. Omega-6 is an essential fatty acid and is normally an important component of cardiovascular health, mental function, and energy production. But when your omega-6 is too high, it can result in inflammation. In every 28 grams (one-ounce serving) peanuts contain 4,000 mg of omega-6.

Peanuts also contain another natural substance called oxalate. When we eat peanuts or peanut butter, and the oxalates become too concentrated in the body's fluids, they will crystallize and lead to health problems. It is recommended that people with gallbladder issues or with untreated or existing kidney problems avoid peanuts altogether. But, for most of us, avoiding peanuts and peanut butter during a detox and then eating it only occasionally is the best plan. I prefer real nut butter like almond butter or cashew butter instead of the butter made from the legume called peanuts.

HIGH GLYCEMIC FRUITS

We want to avoid high-glycemic fruits during a detox because one of our goals is to balance blood sugar and high-glycemic fruits will not help us do this. The higher glycemic fruits are dates, cantaloupe, grapes, raisins, pineapple, and banana. Fruits that are lower on the glycemic index are berries, cherries, apples (especially green apples) and citrus fruits like lemons and limes. These high-glycemic fruits are not unhealthy. They are just higher in natural sugar and should be eliminated, but only during the detox period.

VINEGAR

Avoid vinegar, except organic apple cider vinegar, which is good for many things. The main thing about vinegar is that it makes your body very acidic and one of the goals of the detox is to balance body pH. Organic apple cider vinegar has the opposite effect. Avoid products that contain vinegar, like catsup, mustard, pickles, commercial salad dressings, etc.

WHITE POTATOES

It's not that white potatoes are that bad for you. In fact, they contain many good nutrients and fiber. However, sweet potatoes are a much better choice during a detox because they contain more vitamins, especially vitamin A for eye health, (400% of your daily requirement), and vitamin C for immune system support. Sweet potatoes contain fewer calories, fewer carbs and more fiber than white potatoes.

Both contain potassium and magnesium, but sweet potatoes also contain calcium and manganese, which white potatoes do not. Watch labels when buying sweet potatoes, as yams are not the same thing. They are a cousin of the sweet potato and grow from a different plant. Sweet potatoes have far more nutrients. Believe it or not, white potatoes are higher on the glycemic index (at 70 to 85) than sweet potatoes, which are at 44 on the index.

MEAT

If you choose to eat meat at all, I highly recommend eating the *cleanest* meats you can find. This means grass-fed beef, organic free-range chicken and turkey raised without antibiotics and growth hormones. Grass-fed beef is from cattle that are not fed any GMO corn or other grains and feed only on unsprayed grass pasture. Be aware that some beef claimed to be grass-fed has been "finished" with grain.

Organic free-range chicken, by USDA standards, means the chickens are given access to outdoors. This is loosely enforced. I would recommend locally grown so you can ask the rancher how their chickens and cattle are raised and fed. Of course, I recommend eating as little meat as possible. Besides the toxins in most meat, it is very hard to digest.

PORK

All pork should be avoided during a detox. As for me, I do not eat pork at all. A pig will eat anything and usually does. Pigs do not eliminate toxins in their digestive process or through sweating (pigs don't sweat) and pork contains many dangerous bacteria. It is also possible to get parasites from eating pork.

FISH and SEAFOOD

Farm-raised fish and shrimp should also be avoided because these fish are full of toxins. Tilapia is one of the dirtiest fish you can buy. If buying fish or shrimp, be sure it is wild caught and does not come from China --the waters in China contain nuclear waste from the Fukushima nuclear disaster in Japan, and there is a lack of controls and standards guaranteeing products coming from China are safe.

Summary

Now that we know what to avoid during a detox--gluten, GMO's, dairy, artificial sweeteners, sugar, alcohol and caffeine, bad fats, MSG, vinegar, pork, and processed meats, and farm-raised fish and seafood--what does that leave us to eat, you might ask? In the next chapter, I will give you a plan for what to eat.

Chapter 4

What to Eat During a Detox

We have already determined that we need to give our major detoxing organs time to rid our bodies of toxins and to give our digestive system a rest. In order to do this, we need to consume foods that are easy to digest and have no toxins.

I highly recommend a good protein shake as a meal replacement for one or two meals each day and a clean meal for the third meal of the day, with healthy snacks in between. We also need to improve our gut flora with healthy bacteria and enzymes. A good prebiotic/probiotic is great for this.

Also helpful is to consume a variety of botanicals to support cleansing several ways. Milk thistle and dandelion support the function of the liver and kidneys, important detoxification organs. It is also important to consume antioxidants to help stabilize free radicals and help fight possible oxidative damage. We'll talk about all of these in more detail.

PROTEIN

There are many protein shake mixes on the market, and I have researched just about all of them. So many protein drinks are toxic in themselves. Because there are numerous sources of protein, I want to give you a quick rundown on each kind.

The most common sources of protein in shake mixes and

protein powders on the market today are whey and soy. We have already discussed the dangers of consuming soy. Besides most of the soy being GMO, unfermented soy contains anti-nutrients that keep the body from absorbing the good nutrients. That is totally counterproductive. Soy is not a good option for protein.

Whey is a byproduct of milk. I've covered the many reasons we want to avoid dairy and whey is the part of the cheese making process that is usually discarded. Whey is composed of bovine blood proteins, serum, albumin, lactalbumin, dead white blood cells and hormonal residues including estrogen and progesterone. It is hard to digest, makes your body acidic and can cause many digestive issues. If one of our main goals in a detox is to balance our body's pH, we definitely do not want to consume whey or soy protein.

The best, most easily digested proteins are those from plants like yellow pea, hemp, brown rice, and cranberry seeds. These proteins are easily absorbed by the body, cause no digestive issues and give your body the protein it needs. Avoid protein shake mixes that contain more than 20 grams of protein per serving. The body cannot absorb more than 20 grams at a time. Anything more is overkill. Something else to look for when reading labels on protein shake packages is the sweetener that is used. Many brands use artificial sweeteners like aspartame, which we have already determined should be avoided at all costs. I recommend stevia or monk fruit as a sweetener. These are natural plant-based sweeteners with a low glycemic index and will not cause spikes in blood sugar or add empty calories.

In summary, select a protein shake or powder with a healthy plant-based protein sweetened with stevia or monk fruit.

You will also want to be sure if using a shake mix, that it contains other good nutrients. If it does not contain a well-balanced selection of vitamins and minerals, it shouldn't be used as a meal replacement. Find one that can be made with water or a healthy milk like coconut or almond milk.

A word of caution! If your body is acidic, these shake mixes may not taste great to you. Once your pH is balanced, they will taste much better. To enhance the flavor, you can add organic frozen berries, a tablespoon of almond or cashew butter, cacao, mint or any number of other healthy ingredients. I have included some healthy shake recipes in this chapter.

HEALTHY SNACKS

When detoxing -- and even when not detoxing -- it's important to maintain balanced blood sugar levels. You don't want high and low spikes of blood sugar. You also don't want to get so hungry in between meals that you feel deprived of food and end up eating too much during your meal. So, snacking between meals is a good idea, as long as the snacks are healthy and full of good nutrients.

When you are drinking a protein shake as a meal replacement, you want to be sure to have enough calories. When you don't eat enough calories, your body goes into starvation mode and starts storing fat and burning muscle. So, it's important to take in enough of the right kind of calories; ones that are full of nutrients and not empty calories.

Healthy snacks include raw nuts like almonds, walnuts, pecans, Brazil nuts, and cashews. You will want to avoid peanuts, which aren't a nut at all, but a legume. Peanuts tend to be high in mold and many are allergic to them. Healthy nut butters also make a good snack when paired with gluten-free crackers, rice cakes or vegetables. The most common nut butter is almond butter.

Other good snacks include hummus with vegetables like carrots, celery, jicama or other root vegetables. Lower glycemic fruits such as green apples and berries of any kind are good, too. For these fruits, I would recommend eating organic. When you eat a fruit that doesn't have a rind or a peel, it can contain the most pesticide residue, so it is a good idea to buy organic.

Avocados, guacamole, and salsa that doesn't contain vinegar or sugar are great with a healthy white bean or black bean chip or rice chips. Of course, we want to avoid corn chips, potato chips and any chip fried in canola or other toxic oils. When choosing store-bought snacks, be sure to read labels. Watch out for preservatives, canola, soy, sugars, and ingredients you can't pronounce.

PREBIOTICS and PROBIOTICS

Prebiotics are a soluble fiber on which probiotics feed to stimulate growth. Probiotics are good bacteria that balance out the bad bacteria in your gut. They help with digestion of food and the absorption of nutrients. Probiotics need prebiotics to grow, so it's crucial for a probiotic to also contain a prebiotic.

Examples of prebiotic foods include garlic, onion, leeks, asparagus, apples and dandelion greens. You can also purchase probiotic products that contain prebiotics.

It is also crucial for the probiotic to be one that will survive the acid in the stomach and make it alive to the colon, where it is needed most. Many probiotics on the market will not survive past the stomach.

Probiotic bacteria are measured in CFU's (Colony Forming Units). The more CFU's the better, up to a point. Anything over 40 billion is overkill. Many probiotics also contain enzymes that aid with the breakdown of carbs, fats, protein, fiber, and lactose. Typically, these enzymes are not necessary, as our bodies produce their own digestive enzymes.

But, for someone whose body doesn't make enough digestive enzymes or someone who tends to overeat, additional enzymes can help break down the larger food particles.

Fermented vegetables like sauerkraut and kimchi (both made from cabbage), kombucha and coconut kefir are great for adding good bacteria to your gut. Make your own, or look for brands that contain no sodium benzoate, as this kills the fermentation process.

ANTIOXIDANTS

Antioxidants are molecules that inhibit oxidation of other molecules. They produce enzymes to control free radical chain reactions. Free radicals are a type of highly reactive metabolites which are your body's natural response to environmental toxins. Free radical molecules are missing one or more electrons and this missing electron is responsible for biological oxidation, or biological rusting.

Free radicals steal electrons from the proteins in your body, which badly damages your DNA and other cell structures. Free radicals are linked to over 60 different diseases, including cancer, Parkinson's, Alzheimer's and many others. Antioxidants are electron donors for your cells. They provide your cells with an adequate defense against attack by free radicals.

With these antioxidants, your body can resist aging caused by everyday exposure to pollutants. Antioxidants are important during a detox but are also important every day, to fight off the free radicals from the constant bombardment of environmental toxins.

Examples of antioxidant foods are as follows:

- dark green vegetables – lettuce, leeks, kale, broccoli, collard greens

- sweet potatoes

- red berries

- grapes

- walnuts

- pomegranates

CLEAN EATING

We've talked about drinking two protein meal replacement shakes a day and we've talked about healthy snacks. That leads us to the third aspect of detoxing and that is eating one healthy meal a day. You might be asking "what does 'clean eating' mean"? I already covered the foods to avoid in the last two chapters. So here, I'll cover what you CAN eat!

There are many schools of thought about what clean eating means and there are many different types of diets. By 'diet', I don't mean a temporary diet that you go on to lose weight. By 'diet', I mean the way you eat daily. There are diets like the Paleo diet, which excludes gluten, grains, and most dairy, but includes meat products. Other healthy ways to eat are vegetarian, vegan and raw.

If you choose to eat meat, I recommend a fist-sized portion of grass-fed beef or free-range chicken or turkey and don't eat meat at every meal. In the Standard American Diet (SAD), meat is the focus of the meal. But it really shouldn't be.

My definition of clean eating is mostly plant-based, with an occasional serving of clean meat, if you choose. Include beans, nuts and seeds and plenty of clean water.

If you were to test the American population, you would likely not find many who are deficient in protein. Vegetables and greens should take up 2/3 of your plate. Non-gluten containing whole grains are ok in moderation. These would include brown rice, quinoa or pasta made from these grains. Choose sweet potatoes over white potatoes and eat organic vegetables and fruits whenever possible. We also must not forget healthy fats. Fats are critical to the body. I'll explain more about this. So, let's break it down to make it easier.

Let's talk about gluten first. If you must eat bread, I recommend organic and those made from sprouted grains -- any grains but wheat, barley, and rye. If you want to consume baked goods, there are many flours made from seeds, nuts, and grains besides the ones that contain gluten.

Many supply the body with protein and other necessary nutrients.

Some alternate flours are almond flour, garbanzo bean flour, and brown rice flour, coconut flour, amaranth flour, and oat flour. There are also many gluten-free products on the market that would normally contain gluten. This includes products like pasta, tortillas, granola bars, etc. The best ones are made from the whole grains we mentioned earlier - quinoa, brown rice, amaranth, sorghum, and oats or vegetables like spinach and cauliflower. You might be surprised at what you can make with vegetables, seeds, and nuts.

Many food manufacturers have jumped on the gluten-free bandwagon but be careful of these products. Most are made with GMO Corn unless they are labeled "Organic" or "Non-GMO", so read your labels.

There are also ways to make things like cookies, brownies and other desserts without gluten or sugar. You don't have to skip these yummy treats altogether. I teach some of these recipes and methods in my cooking classes and will include a few recipes at the end of this book.

The best rule of thumb is to stay away from processed foods, processed food products, sugar-laden drinks, basically anything that didn't grow. Eat living foods as much as possible. By "living foods" I mean foods created by God; foods that grow, like fruits, vegetables, clean meats, grains, seeds and nuts.

As far as what to drink, drink the cleanest water you can find. Bottled water isn't often the best choice, but I would choose it over fluoridated, chlorinated tap water if it is the right kind. Many bottled waters are "purified" with chlorine. If you must drink bottled water, choose spring water over "purified" water.

Fluoride is added to city water because it was reported to help prevent cavities. But this has never been proven and fluoride is a known toxin. We'll talk more about this later but know that it is not healthy to ingest fluoride. That's why the toothpaste tube tells you not to swallow your toothpaste. Keep in mind that the fluoride in your toothpaste is absorbed into your body through your tongue, gums and mouth. It is best to use a toothpaste without fluoride.

Chlorine is another known toxin, but the government allows, in fact, mandates 4 parts per million of chlorine in city water. In my opinion, any chlorine is too much and if you can taste it or smell it in the water, that is way too much! Chlorine has been linked to an increase in colon cancer, bladder cancer, asthma, eczema, and heart disease.

I recommend adding citrus to your water, as this is cleansing as well. Lemon juice, lime juice or grapefruit are great options to enhance the flavor and the cleansing properties of your water. Infused water is also good but use organic produce in your infuser. Organic oranges, lemons, limes, mint, and cucumbers are all great options to use in infusing.

Eat lots of low-glycemic fruits like organic green apples and organic berries and lots of vegetables. Vegetables provide you with a multitude of vitamins and minerals along with plenty of necessary fiber. Vegetables don't have many calories, so you can eat as much as you want.

Try to eat all the colors of the rainbow. Purple vegetables like eggplant and purple cabbage; red vegetables like radishes, red peppers and tomatoes; orange vegetables like carrots, sweet potatoes, and orange peppers; and of course, green vegetables like green beans, lima beans, and peas; and leafy green vegetables like cabbage, lettuce, spinach, kale, etc. By eating the rainbow, you are certain to take in all the nutrients you need. Make it a rule to eat at least 2 vegetables with your meal.

Choose organic whenever possible, especially for fruits and vegetables with thin skins or no skin, where you eat the whole thing. Greens, tomatoes, peppers, celery, summer squash like zucchini and yellow squash are all vegetables that should be eaten organic, when possible. The exceptions to this rule are these vegetables that are fairly safe to eat non-organic: asparagus, avocado, cabbage, eggplant, mushrooms, and onions.

If you can't find organic, locally grown is the next best thing. But don't skip your fruits and vegetables just because you can't get organic varieties. Commercially grown is better than nothing.

Consume plenty of healthy fats including nuts, avocado, coconut oil and pure olive oil. Fats are necessary to our bodies because they store energy, insulate us and protect our vital organs. They help proteins do their jobs. They also help control our metabolism by starting chemical reactions that help control growth, immune function, reproduction and other aspects of basic metabolism.

Here, I'd like to share a few words about coconut oil. I believe everyone should have coconut oil in great abundance in their homes. It can be used to cook with, to eat, to clean your teeth, as a moisturizer, as a carrier oil for essential oil use and so many other uses. As far as diet, it acts as an antibacterial and creates a hostile environment for viruses. It contains Lauric acid, which destroys bacteria active in the stomach and the mouth. Interestingly enough, mother's milk contains Lauric acid, which helps immunize infants against infection. The Lauric acid in coconut oil can do the same for adults. Coconut oil also causes the pancreas to produce more insulin, which controls blood sugar. It increases the good cholesterol (HDL) and it contains a healthy fat that converts to energy faster than other fats. It is truly amazing! An entire book could be written about coconut oil. I highly recommend it.

To summarize the 30-day detox period, take a good prebiotic/probiotic, drink two healthy protein shakes and eat a clean meal each day which includes lots of fresh vegetables, healthy fats, and a fist-sized portion of protein, eat a few healthy snacks, drink a detoxing tea containing dandelion or milk thistle, and lots of clean water. Do your detox with a buddy to help you with accountability. I have created an excellent program for anyone who would like day-by-day assistance, recipes, meal ideas and accountability. Contact me through my website at:

www.cleanfoodcleanyou.com

Chapter 5

What to do After Your 30-day Detox

Once you have reset your body, you will want to maintain your clean eating routine as much as possible. The detox should have reduced your cravings for things like carbs, especially sugar.

In this day and age, it's not always possible to eat clean, but some things I recommend you always avoid. Avoid fast food at all costs. Avoid GMO's, processed sugar, bad fats like canola and hydrogenated vegetable oils, and all processed foods. You can re-introduce the higher glycemic fruits but eat them for special treats and not all the time.

If you want to eat some gluten, you can slowly re-introduce gluten-containing foods, but honestly, I would avoid gluten as much as possible. You may find that re-introducing gluten will cause digestive issues for you.

If you have a gluten sensitivity or a gluten intolerance, I would avoid it at all costs. Dairy is the same way. I would limit my intake of dairy because it causes inflammation, mucus and digestion issues.

If you're a cheese-oholic or love ice cream, try limiting your cheese or ice cream intake to special occasions as much as possible or find healthy alternatives. You can make a delicious ice cream with frozen bananas or coconut cream. There are some delicious cheese substitutes made from nuts and other healthy ingredients. See the recipes in the recipes section of the book.

Now that you are equipped with new knowledge about what you're putting in your mouth, be cognizant when you eat, of what you are eating and why.

Besides the taste of the food, be aware of what it is doing for or to your body. Everything you eat is either helping you or hurting you. Get back to the mindset of eating for nourishment and not just for pleasure.

Continue to eat lots of vegetables, clean meats, healthy oils and fats, nuts and seeds and other healthy snacks and substitute healthy desserts for unhealthy ones. I'll give you some ideas for these.

Clean out your pantry of foods that don't serve you. Here are the top 15 things you can do to clean out your pantry and start your journey to a healthier you. Don't worry if you can't do this all at once. Baby steps will get you miles ahead.

1. Replace canola oil or other hydrogenated vegetable oils, including margarine, with coconut oil, extra virgin olive oil, and avocado oil. Cook with coconut oil and use olive oil in salad dressings and low-heat cooking. Make your own salad dressings. I have found that many commercial dressings on the market use hydrogenated oils, especially soy and canola oil, as well as high fructose corn syrup and other sweeteners. Choose a vegan butter or organic butter instead of margarine or make a nut butter from cashews.

2. Replace processed sugar with healthier sweeteners. Use coconut sugar or organic cane sugar if you must use sugar at all. Use pure

maple syrup, honey, stevia or monk fruit for sweetening oatmeal, natural pudding (I'll share this recipe with you) and other foods. Find recipes for desserts that sweeten with sweet fruits like dates, prunes, currants, dried coconut, and raisins.

3. Replace bromated flour with healthier flour. If you don't want to give up gluten, I would recommend unbleached, un-bromated, organic wheat flour. If you want to be gluten-free, there are many bean or seed flours, as I mentioned above.

4. Eat brown rice instead of bleached white rice or substitute quinoa or lentils for rice once in a while. And you don't have to give up your pasta. Choose brown rice or quinoa pasta instead of wheat. Better yet, have some spaghetti squash spaghetti or spiralized zucchini noodles. There are all sorts of options.

5. When it comes to something crunchy, choose white bean or black bean chips instead of GMO corn chips. They taste great with a healthy salsa! Buy gluten-free crackers (just read the labels and watch for hydrogenated oils and GMO corn). Buy sweet potato chips (baked not fried) or make your own! These are super easy to make.

6. Choose alternative milks. Instead of dairy milk, try unsweetened almond milk, coconut milk or cashew milk. Read the ingredients here, too.

Watch out for sweeteners and carrageenan and avoid milk with these ingredients or other additives.

7. Instead of bleached table salt, buy pink Himalayan sea salt or other healthy sea salts. These come full of healthy minerals your body needs.

8. Buy organic apple cider vinegar instead of other vinegar. It has a million uses and provides excellent health benefits.

9. Choose natural maple syrup instead of the artificially flavored, high fructose corn syrup fakes on the market. It's more expensive, but your health is worth the extra cost! Because of its purity, you don't need to use as much.

10. Buy organic eggs or use a flax egg as a substitute, if you'd like to eat Vegan, when making recipes like pancakes, waffles, cookies, quick breads and muffins. A flax egg is 1 tablespoon of ground flax seed mixed with 2.5 tablespoons of water. Let sit for 5 minutes to thicken.

11. Drink clean water instead of pop or other sweetened drinks and drink from a glass or stainless-steel container. Add a drop of grapefruit, lemon, lime, or orange essential oil to your water or a squeeze of lemon or lime juice.

NOTE: You do not want to add essential oils to water in a plastic bottle or container. Essential oils will pull petrochemicals from plastic. Use glass or stainless steel. When using essential oils, be sure to buy top-quality oils with nutrition facts listed on the bottle. Unless they have nutrition facts, they are not safe to ingest. Infused waters are great, too, but choose organic fruit, if at all possible, and wash the rinds of citrus fruits before you use them for this purpose.

12. Choose a natural almond butter or cashew butter instead of peanut butter. As I mentioned before, peanut butter tends to contain mold, and most are sweetened with sugar or corn syrup. Nut butters are easy to make at home, especially if you have a food processor. Just put oven roasted nuts in the food processor and blend.

13. Have a healthy shake for breakfast, or oatmeal or chia pudding, instead of a heavy breakfast of meat, gluten, and eggs or a sugary processed cereal, toaster pastry or donut. Add some frozen organic strawberries or blueberries to your shake. When your bananas start to turn brown, instead of throwing them away, peel them and break them in half and freeze for use in your morning shake.

14. For snacks, instead of processed food products from the vending machines, choose organic berries, apples, carrots or nuts and seeds like walnuts, almonds, pecans, sunflower seeds

(unprocessed, of course), or dried fruit, as long as it doesn't have nitrates or nitrites, other chemical preservatives or added sugar.

15. Purchase fresh or frozen vegetables over canned, whenever possible. Most canned vegetables have added salt and can absorb chemicals from the can, especially if the can is lined with plastic. Look for BPA-free cans.

I can't stress enough, READ LABELS and avoid ingredients you can't pronounce. Watch out for labels that say things like "Natural" or "Gluten-Free", "low-fat" or "fat-free". Often, these products contain chemically derived ingredients, GMO corn or processed ingredients.

Know that when a label says "Non-GMO" that is not the same thing as organic. But if a food is organic, it is also Non-GMO. Learning to replace bad ingredients with good ones can make a huge difference to your health.

It just takes some thought and preparation. Read labels and find good healthy brands and stick to those brands. This makes shopping easier. Shop the outside aisles of the store and skip the inner aisles as much as possible. This is where all the processed food is shelved.

Make your health a priority and you will have a much longer, more enjoyable life. I will include some recipes later in this book to help you get started on your journey to a healthier you. And it is a journey. Don't be too hard on yourself. Take it one day at a time. If you can get to the point where you can eat healthy 80% of the time, you will be much healthier, will feel better and can skate into old age with no issues!

In chapter 8, I'll teach you what toxic chemicals are lurking in the products you use every day on your hair and body and what you can do to eliminate these toxins. But first, let's look at supplements.

Chapter 6

Supplements

The subject of supplements is a big one and an entire book could be written on it. Many people in the healthy eating arena will tell you that due to the poor quality of our food nowadays, our food provides only *supplemental* nutrition and supplements have become our main source of nutrients. There are so many superfood nutrients emerging, it's hard to know what to take and what not to take.

Doctors who have studied this subject have determined that most people are deficient in several nutrients that are vital to the human body. We'll talk about some of these many people may not think about.

IODINE

One of these nutrients is Iodine. Every cell in the body contains iodine. The thyroid gland contains the highest concentration of iodine. Large amounts are also stored in the breasts and ovaries and in the brain.

Iodine is found in many foods from the sea, such as saltwater fish like cod, sea bass and haddock and in sea vegetables like seaweed. Because most of us don't live near an ocean and don't eat a lot of seafood and because much of our seafood is tainted due to the toxins in our oceans, up to 95% of people are iodine deficient.

The U.S. government determined that a good way to provide people with more iodine was to add it to table salt. But the salt they added it to is devoid of all the minerals salt usually provides our bodies and the amount of iodine we get from eating the salt is not enough to supply the body's needs.

The bioavailability of iodine in salt has been shown to be only 10%. Just a few of the conditions that can be treated with iodine are breast diseases, thyroid disorders, ovarian diseases, fatigue, headaches, including migraines and prostate disorders. Iodine supplementation can be accomplished by taking Iodoral or Lugol's solution. It is recommended to consult with your healthcare practitioner before taking iodine supplements, as dosages vary and too much iodine can be detrimental.

VITAMIN C

Vitamin C is a water-soluble vitamin important in its role as an antioxidant and for maintaining the health of the body's connective tissue. Some of the benefits of vitamin C include strengthening the immune system, protecting against cardiovascular disease, prenatal health problems, eye disease, and skin wrinkling.

We need to ingest vitamin C daily in order to maintain necessary supplies. Our body does not produce vitamin C and doesn't store it. So, we need to replenish vitamin C in our bodies every day. Good sources of vitamin C are fruits and vegetables.

The fruits and vegetables with the most Vitamin C are listed in order of potency here. It is best to consume these foods fresh and raw to get the most benefit. Guava, black currant, red bell pepper, kiwi, green bell pepper, oranges, strawberries, papaya, broccoli, kale, parsley, pineapple,

Brussels sprouts, grapefruit, peas, cauliflower, and mango. Consuming 2 to 3 of these vitamin C rich foods daily will help you maintain proper levels.

VITAMIN D

Another nutrient many people are deficient in is vitamin D. The reason most people don't get enough vitamin D is that we tend to spend too much time indoors and we slather ourselves with sunscreen when we do go outside.

There aren't many foods that naturally contain vitamin D and fortified foods, like milk, don't provide our bodies with enough. The main food group that contains vitamin D are fatty fish such as wild-caught salmon, tuna, and mackerel and fish liver oil. Vitamin D is not actually a vitamin, but a steroid hormone that our bodies were designed to get from sun exposure.

Increasing levels of vitamin D3 could prevent chronic diseases that claim nearly one million lives throughout the world each year. Optimizing your vitamin D levels may help you prevent cancer, heart disease, autoimmune diseases, infections, mental health conditions, and more.

Studies show it reduces the risk of colorectal cancer, prostate cancer, and a whole host of other deadly cancers by 30 to 50 percent. Vitamin D also fights infections, including colds and the flu. It is an extremely important nutrient and any doctor can test you for a deficiency.

Vitamin D supplementation should be paired with vitamin K2, but if you get your vitamin D from the sun, you don't need to worry about that. A good way to judge the length of time you need in the sun to get enough vitamin D is by judging the length of time it takes you to get sunburned. If you get sunburned after 30 minutes in the sun, you should be getting enough vitamin D after 15 minutes. Keep in mind that in order to absorb vitamin D from the sun, your skin has to be exposed to the sun. It's not sufficient to just be outside if you are covered up by clothing.

OMEGA-3 FATTY ACIDS

Omega-3 fatty acids are important in reducing inflammation, and as we've already discussed in chapter 1, this is vitally important in preventing many diseases, as most disease in the body stems from inflammation.

Many people are deficient in omega-3's because of the prevalence of omega-6 fatty acids consumed in processed foods and hydrogenated oils. The proper ratio for omega-6's vs omega-3's should be 2 to 1. But most Americans have a ratio of 20 to 1.

Like vitamin D, omega-3 is only found in a few food sources. The best sources of the healthiest form of omega-3 is, interestingly enough, the same food sources of vitamin D: wild caught salmon, sardines, and mackerel.

Other sources, in order of available omega-3, are grass-fed beef, flaxseed, chia seed, walnuts, and tuna. Other high omega-3 foods include Brussels sprouts, cauliflower, and seaweed.

There are lots of omega-3 supplements on the market, including fish oil, but be careful what you purchase. Many fish oil supplements are rancid or contain high levels of toxins due to their sourcing. Do your research and read labels if you choose to take a fish oil supplement. Use caution in selecting your tuna, as well. Many brands of tuna contain high levels of mercury, which is extremely toxic.

CHLORELLA

Chlorella is a supplement I recommend for everyone. It is a cracked cell wall single-cell green algae -- an amazing source of nutrition. Chlorella is high in zinc, iron, magnesium, vitamins C, E, and B12. Chlorella boosts your energy, supports fat loss and helps detox heavy metals like lead and mercury from your body. You can take it in tablet form or add the powder to a shake.

TURMERIC

Turmeric is a yellow spice from India. It can be used in many dishes, as it doesn't have a strong flavor. Turmeric has many healing properties, most of which come from curcumin contained in turmeric. It is a strong antioxidant. Not only does it kill free radicals in your body, but it stimulates your body to create its own antioxidant enzymes.

It also reduces inflammation and increases brain health by increasing the growth of new neurons in the brain. Turmeric is beneficial to your whole body. I recommend a good curcumin extract, turmeric essential oil or, at the very least, using turmeric in your cooking.

GINGER

Ginger is a flowering plant originating in China. The part of the ginger plant used as a spice is the rhizome, or root, the part of the stem that grows underground. It is well known for helping with digestion and nausea, but it also helps fight flu and cold viruses.

The nausea fighting capabilities of ginger go way back. Ginger was used to relieve seasickness. It has also been shown to be effective in helping to relieve morning sickness, nausea after surgery and in cancer patients undergoing chemotherapy.

Other uses for ginger include helping to lower blood sugar levels, reducing joint pain and muscle pain. It can be added to smoothies, taken as a supplement or used in cooking and baking. It can be purchased in powder form, as an oil or juice, crystallized or raw.

MACA

Maca is a cruciferous vegetable. It is native to Peru and only grows in high altitudes. The edible part of the plant is the root. It is highly nutritious and is a great source of several important vitamins. One ounce of Maca contains 4 grams of protein, vitamin C, iron, potassium, vitamin B6 and manganese. It has been known to reduce symptoms of menopause, improve mood, reduce anxiety, increase energy and improve brain function, including learning and memory, and may enhance fertility. It can be purchased at health food stores or online in powder form and can be added to shakes and smoothies, oatmeal or just about anything. It adds a nice caramel malt-like flavor.

Chapter 7

Cooking Methods

I want to include a short section here on cooking methods, because the research I read has found that this definitely matters to your health.

I recommend eating raw fruits and vegetables as much as possible. If you choose to cook them, steaming is the best way, as the most nutrients are retained with this method. Boiling, unless you drink the water used to boil the vegetables, leaches out much of the nutrients. I caution you, however, to not over-cook your vegetables. They should remain firm and not mushy. The less time you cook vegetables, the more nutrients they retain.

As far as what pots and pans to use, there are differing opinions. As it is my position to avoid as many unnecessary toxins in my life as possible, I avoid using aluminum pans and copper pans due to the leaching of these metals into your food. It has been said that aluminum can be tied to Alzheimer's. The same goes for using aluminum foil. More of the metal is leached into the food when the pot or pan is pitted and worn and when cooking acidic foods, such as tomatoes. Don't store food in aluminum.

The best pans are Cast Iron, Stainless Steel and glass. Cast Iron can actually provide some of the iron we all need in our diets. I haven't done any research on the new Granite non-stick pans, but I would think these would be a good choice. Ceramic is also fine but doesn't tend to hold up very well.

Plastic should be eliminated as much as possible. Many plastic containers and can liners contain BPA, bisphenol A. This chemical is a synthetic estrogen and has been linked to many health problems. Look for BPA free cans and plastic containers and bottles. Store food in glass containers whenever possible.

When it comes to heating or cooking food, there has been much controversy. Is the microwave safe or not? Should you microwave in plastic or not? Again, I have read the research on this and it is my opinion that like Roundup, processed food products, hydrogenated oils and many other things that have been proven to be detrimental to our health, the government has chosen to sweep these studies under the rug in the name of profits. There have been studies that date back as far as the early 1990's that show the dangers of exposing our food to microwave radiation.

There was a case in 1991 of a lawsuit in Oklahoma. A woman named Norma Levitt had hip surgery and needed a blood transfusion. A nurse warmed the blood for the transfusion in a microwave oven. The results, the patient died! It is quite apparent that there is more to 'heating' with microwaves than we've been led to believe. In the case of Mrs. Levitt, the microwaving altered the blood and it killed her. Does this make you think that this form of heating does, indeed, do 'something different' to the substances being heated?

There have also been studies done with plants being watered with microwaved water vs filtered water. You can read about this at the link below. Suffice it to say the plants watered with microwaved water did poorly, or died, while the plants watered with filtered water thrived.

https://www.cwgministries.org/blogs/does-microwaved-water-effect-plant-growth-my-grandchildren-did-research-project

You might wonder why heating with the microwave oven is any different than heating on the stove or other conventional methods. Conventional heating warms the food by transferring heat from the outside to the inside.

Microwaves, on the other hand, heat food very differently. A scientist from Switzerland, Hans Hertel, has this explanation about how microwaves work. "Atoms, molecules and cells hit by this hard electromagnetic radiation are forced to reverse polarity 1 to 100 billion times a second. There are no atoms, molecules or cells of any organic system able to withstand such a violent, destructive power for any extended period of time, not even in the low energy range of milliwatts. Of all the natural substances-which are polar-the oxygen of water molecules reacts most sensitively. This is how microwave cooking heat is generated-friction from this violence in water molecules. Structures of molecules are torn apart, molecules are forcefully deformed (called structural isomerism) and thus become impaired in quality."

The results of ingesting foods that have been altered in this way, are changes in the body and blood that mimic changes that occur with high stress situations. These changes include high cholesterol, an increase in white blood cells, decreased hemoglobin and other detrimental blood changes.

With all of this information that has been suppressed for years, why are microwaves even still on the market? Wouldn't you rather take a few extra minutes to heat something on the stove or in the oven than to alter your food or drink in such a way as to damage your body in this way?

I choose not to use the microwave. Of course, the decision is up to you.

Section 3

Your Environment

Chapter 8

Toxins in Personal Care Products

In this chapter, I'm going to talk about the toxins we absorb through our largest organ, our skin. Everything you put on your skin, including in your mouth, is absorbed by your body in approximately 30 seconds.

Most people think that if they sell it in the store, it must be safe for us to use. Right? If it's in the baby aisle and marketed for babies, it must be gentle and safe. Right? This is oh-so-wrong.

Most of the personal care products sold in the big discount stores are anything but safe or gentle. Products we use every day -- without even thinking about them --are putting harmful toxins in our bodies and in our children's bodies.

The EPA and FDA will tell you these products are safe because they only contain "a little bit" of these toxic ingredients. But when you combine multiple products each day and use them every day and sometimes multiple times per day, the effects are multiplied hundreds of times over.

When you stop to think about all the products you use daily, especially women, you will see that you are increasing your toxic load every day. Most everyone uses toothpaste at least once or twice a day and deodorant or antiperspirant at least once a day.

Then there are shampoo and conditioner, body wash, facial cleanser, facial moisturizer, body moisturizer, perfume, makeup of all sorts, anti-aging products, eye cream, nail polish, hair dye, powders, and soaps. The list is endless.

Most women use at least 10 products on their bodies every day. Below is a partial list of toxic ingredients to avoid when using all these products. I have listed them in alphabetical order for easy reference.

The key is to learn to recognize these ingredients and read labels when purchasing products. Many "natural" lines will contain some healthy, natural ingredients, but will also contain some of these chemical toxins.

It is safest to make your own using naturally occurring ingredients. But if you don't want to do that, there are healthy options available. I stay away from all the cosmetics, hair care products, body products, toothpaste, and deodorant at drug stores and discount stores and either make my own, purchase healthier products at health food stores or buy online from reputable companies. You just can't find healthy products at these stores. The prices are cheap for a reason. They contain cheap, toxic ingredients I will not use on my body or on my children.

Aluminum - Aluminum is a metal, which is used in antiperspirants. It helps to keep you "dry" by blocking the sweat from escaping the pores. Aluminum has been linked to breast cancer in women and has also been linked to an increased risk of Alzheimer's disease.

Our bodies sweat to release toxins and to cool our bodies. It is not healthy to block the pores from releasing the sweat and the toxins. There are better ways to keep from offending.

There are many healthier alternatives to the toxic deodorants and antiperspirants found in most stores. There are many brands found in health food stores and online that are all natural and contain none of these toxins. You can also use a natural crystal deodorant or make your own with essential oils.

Behentrimonium Chloride - Behentrimonium chloride is a type of ammonium salt used as a preservative and surfactant. It is a toxic compound, with concentrations of 0.1% and higher having been shown to damage the eyes. It is irritating to the skin and causes inflammation.

Cocamidopropyl Betaine - This foaming agent has been associated with skin and eye irritation and allergic contact dermatitis. Although the government regards it as safe, many people have negative reactions to it.

Diethanolamine (DEA), TEA (Triethanolamine) and MEA (Monoethanolamine) - These substances are harsh solvents and detergents that are used in cosmetics and face and body creams as an emollient. They can cause allergic reactions, and long-term use of DEA-based products (such as Cocamide DEA) have been linked to an increase in the incidence of liver and kidney cancer.

Dimethicone - Dimethicone is a silicone oil that can make the scalp and skin incredibly dry and irritated. It forms an almost plastic-like barrier on the outside of the skin and traps bacteria, sebum, and impurities with it. It is also an eye irritant and is non-biodegradable and horrible for the environment.

Fluoride - The active ingredient in toothpaste is listed as sodium fluoride. Fluoride is a toxic halogen element. It has not been proven to prevent cavities and it says on the tube "do not swallow". Even if you don't swallow it, you are absorbing it through your gums and tongue.

Answer me this. If you are not supposed to swallow fluoride, why then, do they put toxic fluoride in city water? The goal was to reduce tooth decay, but this has never been proven to work. Fluoridated water has caused more issues than it has solved. If you can, avoid drinking fluoridated water and using fluoride toothpaste.

There are brands of toothpaste that do not have this toxin and there are recipes to make your own and save you some money in the process. A mixture of baking soda, water and a drop of an essential oil like peppermint will do the trick. Add some food-grade bentonite clay for even more cleaning and whitening.

Fragrance - Beware of a product that lists "fragrance" as an ingredient. Chemical fragrance of any kind clogs the lymphatic system and induces major organ system toxicity. They also cause endocrine disruption. There are hundreds of natural essential oils that can give you an unlimited number of different smells for shampoo and conditioner and other body products. The citrus oils are especially nice for this.

Isopropyl Alcohol - Isopropyl alcohol is used as a solvent in many skin care products. It causes skin irritation and strips the skin of its natural acid mantle, promoting the growth of bacteria, molds, and viruses. It may also cause premature aging of the skin.

Mineral Oil - Mineral oil is derived from petroleum (crude oil). It is commonly found as the main ingredient of face and body creams and cosmetics. Baby oil is 100% mineral oil! It coats the skin like a plastic film, clogging pores and stopping the skin from eliminating toxins, which can lead to acne and other skin disorders. If you put a cracker in a container of mineral oil, it will not dissolve, as you would expect. Instead, it becomes hard as a rock and will last forever! Try it!! Other petroleum-based ingredients include paraffin wax, paraffin oil, and petrolatum.

Parabens - Parabens are a chemical compound of para-hydroxybenzoic acid, and they are used as preservatives. Most that are added to our cosmetics are man-made and not naturally occurring. They are often found in deodorants and are widely used in cosmetics, skin care, and baby products to prolong their shelf life.

A random sampling of 100 human urine specimens performed by the CDC showed that all 100 contained parabens. This demonstrates the high absorption rate of chemicals we place on our skin.

Recent scientific studies in the UK found a strong link between the use of parabens and the increasing rate of breast cancer in women. Researchers found a high concentration of parabens in 90% of breast tumors tested.

Phenoxyethanol - Another preservative used in cosmetics and hair care products. It causes organ system toxicity and is an irritant to the skin, eyes, and lungs. The FDA even warned that phenoxyethanol can cause shut down of the central nervous system, vomiting and contact dermatitis.

Phthalates - Pronounced "tha-late," phtalates are another class of chemicals that are often used in deodorants and antiperspirants that you will want to avoid. Phthalates are used in cosmetics, synthetic fragrances, plastics, body care products, and medical goods. They help to dissolve other ingredients and to create a better consistency. The problem with phthalates is that they have been linked to a variety of health issues. High thallate blood and urine levels in women of childbearing age have been linked to a higher risk of birth defects. This suggests that phthalates may disrupt hormone receptors as well as increase the likelihood of cell mutation.

Polyethylene Glycol (PEG) - PEG *is* often found in conditioners and is used as a thickener in skin care products and cosmetics. PEG contains dangerous dioxin levels, often found as a byproduct of the ethoxylation process in manufacturing. Dioxins have a direct link to cancer and cause organ system toxicity. PEGs interfere with the skin's natural moisture balance, causing an increase in aging and leaving the skin vulnerable to bacteria.

Polysorbates - These are used to dissolve fragrance or other oil additives. Often found in conditioners. It leaves a residue on the skin and scalp, disrupts the skin's natural pH and destroys the natural protective barrier of our skin and scalp. Polysorbate-80 is the worst of the bunch – but steer clear of all!

Potassium Sorbate - Potassium sorbate is used as a preservative in hair care products. It causes skin and organ system toxicity.

Propylene Glycol - Propylene glycol is another common ingredient that is used in antiperspirants and deodorants. This is a petroleum-based material that is used to soften cosmetic products due to its slick consistency. It is a cheap way to make skin care products more easily applied to the skin. It causes skin rashes and contact dermatitis and has been shown to cause damage to the kidneys and liver.

Quaternium-15 - This lovely chemical is another quaternary ammonium salt used as a surfactant and preservative in personal care products. It acts as a formaldehyde releaser and is not safe. Formaldehyde is extremely carcinogenic and should be avoided at all costs.

Retinyl Palmitate - Retinyl palmitate, a form of vitamin A, can speed the development of skin tumors and lesions, making it a possible carcinogen. It causes reproductive toxicity and organ system toxicity.

Sodium Lauryl Sulfate/Sodium Laureth Sulfate (SLS) and Ammonium Lauryl Sulfate (ALS) - These ingredient are surfactants found in many cleaning products, shampoos, toothpaste, foaming facial and body cleansers and bubble bath. It is also classified as an insecticide.

The sodium and ammonium laureate sulfates are known cancer-causing ingredients that can cause liver damage, skin rashes, depression, diarrhea, and eye damage. They are easily absorbed into the body, building up in the brain, heart, lungs, and liver, leading to potential long-term health problems. SLS and ALS may also cause cataracts and prevent children's eyes from developing properly.

Talc - Talc is a soft mineral used in talcum powders, including baby powder, and cosmetic powders. Scientific studies have shown that routine application of talcum powder to the genital area is linked with a three- to fourfold increase in the development of ovarian cancer. Inhaling cosmetic powders containing talc may also be harmful to long-term health.

Triclosan - Triclosan is another common ingredient included in commercial deodorants, shampoos and conditioners. It is utilized as the odor killing part of antiperspirants for its anti-bacterial properties. It is also commonly used in antibacterial soaps, hand wipes, and gels. Triclosan is classified as a pesticide by the FDA.

It can accumulate in our fat cells and keep our body in a state of toxicity. It causes irritation of the skin, eyes, and lungs, and causes endocrine disruption and organ system toxicity. It is classified as a probable carcinogen by the Environmental Protection Agency. This classification has prompted some companies to remove it from their products. However, it still can be found as an ingredient in some formulas.

Remember, if you can't pronounce it, it's probably not good for you. Read labels, clean out your medicine cabinet and bathroom cabinets and replace those toxic products you are using every day on yourself and your children. If a major change is not possible for you right now, just start with replacing one product a week or one product a month and make some of your own products. Check out products you are considering at the Environmental Working Group's website at:

www.ewg.org

Chapter 9

Green Cleaning

Where do I start with this subject! There are whole books written on green cleaning, so just know this: there has always been dirt and grime, germs, fungus, viruses, and bacteria. There ARE natural safe ways to take care of all these things. Something else to consider is that our bodies are made up of more good and bad bacteria than anything else. We don't need to live in a completely sterile environment. A little dirt and germs help to strengthen our immune systems.

The products on the store shelves are full of chemicals that are toxic to you, your children and your pets. Not only do they contain toxins you are taking in on your skin (unless you are wearing rubber gloves, some of those are toxic, too), but you are also breathing in those toxic fumes.

Have you ever read the back of those bottles of household cleaners? They usually recommend that you don't breathe them (how do you avoid that?) and that you use gloves. Why is that? They are dangerous. There are easily obtained, natural ingredients that are cheaper and safer to use and are just as effective. A few of my favorites are listed below.

Bathroom Cleaning Powder

Instead of the bleach-filled toxic cleaning powder you buy at the store, combine these ingredients and store in a mason jar or a large empty spice container.

2 cups borax

1 cup baking soda

¼ cup kosher salt

10 drops melaleuca essential oil

10 drops lemon essential oil

To use, dampen the surface to be cleaned with water or white vinegar and sprinkle the cleaning powder over the area. Let sit for 10 to 15 minutes and scrub with a sponge or brush. Rinse clean.

Multi-purpose Cleaning Spray

Use this spray to clean kitchen countertops, porcelain, glass or tile.

1 cup distilled white vinegar or organic apple cider vinegar

2 cups distilled water

5 drops melaleuca essential oil

5 drops lemon essential oil

Add ingredients to a 12 oz glass spray bottle. Shake well.

Some ingredients commonly used in green cleaning products are salt, white vinegar or organic apple cider vinegar, baking soda, borax, castile soap, and essential oils. I highly recommend essential oils as part of a healthy home transformation. Melaleuca kills bacteria, viruses, and fungus. The citrus essential oils have constituents that have antifungal, antibacterial and antiseptic properties, so these are excellent oils for cleaning. Besides all that, they have a wonderful clean aroma. These ingredients, in the right combinations, will clean just about anything.

Take a day to detox your home of toxic cleaning products. Replace your bathroom cleaners, kitchen cleaners, window and floor cleaners, laundry products and dish soaps with these simple, inexpensive recipes. If you can't bring yourself to throw away what you have, just use it up and instead of buying more of the toxic products, decide to replace it with a clean recipe. Check out my blog for more green cleaning recipes at:

https://www.cleanfoodcleanyou.com/blog

Something else to consider - skip the "air freshener" and chemical-filled candles. Have you noticed how candle fragrances are chemical versions of natural smells, like lemon, cinnamon, lavender, rose, etc? And these chemical fakes don't smell as good as the real thing. Invest in a diffuser and diffuse the natural essential oils from the real plant. They will smell better, clean your air and won't clog your lungs with toxic chemical fragrance. A great resource for recipes to make your own healthy body care and cleaning products is The Smart Mom's Guide to Essential Oils, by Dr. Mariza Snyder.

Essential Oils and Health

I wanted to say a bit more about essential oils. They have powerful constituents that can help with so many things. Again, an entire book could be written, and has, about the benefits and uses of essential oils.

I have found that essential oils can replace many over-the-counter remedies for everyday issues. Oils like oregano, melaleuca, and thyme are amazing antifungal, anti-bacterial, and anti-viral. There are blends of oils that can help reduce colds and flu. There are oils like lavender and ylang-ylang for calming nervousness, irritability, and restlessness. There are oils that can help you sleep, wake you up or improve your brain function. There are oils that can soothe an upset stomach, achy joints and muscles, and headache.

As an example, one client of mine had leg pains due to arthritis that kept her up at night. She started using 1 drop of frankincense mixed with a healthy body lotion on the bottoms of her feet at night. Her leg pains ceased, and she was able to sleep better and move better in the morning.

There are essential oils that can soothe bug bites, rashes, toothaches, acne, and other skin issues. They can help reduce the fine lines of aging, dry skin and age spots.

In short, essential oils can help with so many things. I highly recommend them and can provide guidance about their use. Contact me through my website at:

www.cleanfoodcleanyou.com

Section 4

This and That

Chapter 10

Health Care Options

You might be thinking that it's all well and good to eat healthy, rid our bodies of toxins and use natural products and essential oils, but what do we do if we get really sick?

It has been my experience that most minor illnesses can be treated with supplements and essential oils, but some of us have health issues that have been forming in our bodies for many years. That's why I encourage young people to start early to take care of themselves; so serious illness doesn't rear its ugly head when we get older.

But what do we do if we get really sick? I will honestly tell you that I am not a fan of conventional medicine when it comes to most illness. Through no fault of their own, medical doctors are trained to treat symptoms with pills. Most medications are toxins in and of themselves. If you listen to drug commercials on TV, you know that often the side effects of taking the drugs, are more numerous and more dangerous than the benefits.

I will say that for trauma, the U.S. medical system is the best. I would so go to the doctor or the hospital if I were in a car accident or broke my arm or had a burst appendix. But for illness, I choose a more natural practitioner trained in nutrition.

So here I'd like to explain the different types of alternative health practitioners, as this can be very confusing.

Functional Medicine Practitioner is one who seeks to identify and address the root causes of disease and views the body as one integrated system, not a collection of independent organs divided up by medical specialties. They treat the whole system, not just the symptoms. The best functional medicine practitioners are ones who studied conventional medicine and then pursued more education in nutrition and natural treatments.

Holistic Medicine Practitioner is a practitioner who considers the whole person – body, mind, spirit, and emotions – in the quest for optimal health and wellness. Holistic practitioners believe that, if people have imbalances (physical, emotional, or spiritual) in their lives, it can negatively affect their overall health.

Holistic medicine is an umbrella term used to describe a variety of therapies that attempt to treat the patient as a whole person.

Homeopathy is a type of holistic medicine but has a distinctly unique approach compared to other types of holistic medicine, like naturopathic medicine or traditional Chinese medicine.

Integrative Medicine may refer to physicians, physical therapists, and psychological counselors. There may be an emphasis on nutrition and wellness, or diet and supplements, but the medical component of an integrative medicine clinic is often along the lines of conventional medicine using drugs to counter symptoms. Generally, integrated physicians fail to delve deeply into the factors that are keeping their patients from realizing a true state of health.

Naturopathic Doctors (NDs) are general practitioners of natural medicine. They are trained to treat ailments using clinical nutrition, acupuncture, botanical medicine, physical medicine, lifestyle counseling, and homeopathy.

Naturopathic medicine is a distinct primary health care profession, emphasizing prevention, treatment, and optimal health using therapeutic methods and substances which encourage the person's inherent self-healing process.

Homeopathic Medicine is the practice of medicine that embraces a holistic, natural approach to the treatment of the sick. Homeopathy is holistic because it treats the person, rather than focusing on a diseased part or a labeled sickness.

Homeopathy believes a substance that causes the symptoms of a disease in healthy people would cure similar symptoms in sick people.

I highly recommend alternative forms of health care when necessary. Do your research to find someone you can trust.

Most insurance companies don't pay for alternative forms of health care, yet. There are a few groups that do, but most of the time you'll have to pay out of pocket for this type of treatment. In my opinion, it's worth every penny.

Chapter 11

RECIPES

Desserts

Banana Ice Cream

3 large ripe bananas – peeled and cut into pieces and frozen

½ teaspoon cinnamon

½ teaspoon vanilla

Pinch of sea salt

Toppings – fresh fruit, coconut, cacao nibs, nuts or seeds.

Let bananas soften at room temperature for about 5 minutes. Combine bananas, cinnamon, vanilla, and salt in a blender. Blend until smooth and creamy. Pour into a bowl, mix in your favorite toppings and serve immediately, or add to Popsicle molds and freeze for later.

Coconut Cream Ice Cream

2 cups full-fat canned coconut milk

¼ cup maple syrup

Pinch of monk fruit sweetener, coconut sugar or stevia

1/8 teaspoon salt

1 teaspoon pure vanilla extract

Place all ingredients in a large bowl and stir together. If using an ice cream maker, transfer the mixture to your ice cream maker and proceed using manufacturer's directions.

If you don't have an ice cream maker, freeze the mixture in the bowl or use ice trays. If using ice trays, blend frozen cubes with a high-speed blender until creamy. If using the bowl, freeze for 30 minutes, remove from the freezer and beat with a mixer or immersion blender. Return to the freezer. Repeat these steps until ice cream is creamy and frozen.

Chocolate Thumbprint Cookies

½ cup almond flour

½ cup gluten-free oats

½ cup garbanzo bean flour

3 tablespoons cacao powder

½ teaspoon pink Himalayan sea salt

¼ cup coconut oil

¼ cup pure maple syrup

1 teaspoon vanilla

Fruit sweetened jam of your choice (apricot, cherry, raspberry, strawberry)

Preheat oven to 350 degrees. Place the oats into a food processor and pulse until ground. Combine almond flour, oat flour, garbanzo bean flour, cacao, and salt into a large bowl and stir to combine. Add melted coconut oil, maple syrup, and vanilla. Stir to combine. Roll a tablespoon of dough into a ball in your hands and place 2 inches apart on a baking sheet. Make an indentation in the center of each cookie with your thumb. Spoon a teaspoon of jam into the center. Bake cookies for 15 minutes. Transfer to a rack to cool for 10 minutes.

Store in an airtight container. Cookies will keep for several days.

Dessert Crepes

1 tablespoon organic butter – melted

1 Egg

½ cup almond or coconut milk

½ cup gluten-free all-purpose flour

½ teaspoon organic sugar or honey

Pinch of sea salt

¾ cup fresh or frozen berries or cut fruit (blueberries, strawberries, pineapple, raspberries, mango, banana, peaches)

Pour all ingredients, except fruit, into a blender, food processor or bowl. Combine until smooth. If using a bowl, a whisk is recommended. Heat a crepe pan or other non-stick skillet to med-high. Wipe the hot pan with a little butter or coconut oil. Pour about ½ cup of the batter into the pan, just to coat the bottom. Quantity will vary depending on the size of your pan. Rotate and tip the pan to spread the batter. Cook until the batter moves loosely around the pan – about 1 minute. Flip the crepe over and cook another minute. Remove from pan to a plate. Place fruit in the pan and stir just to warm the fruit. Put the fruit on the crepe and fold into a triangle or roll it up. Top with powdered sugar or whipped cream, if desired.

Raw Chocolate Pudding, a healthy pudding you can eat for breakfast

  1 ripe banana

  1 ripe avocado

  4 Tablespoons cacao powder

  ½ teaspoon allspice

  1 teaspoon vanilla

  2 Tablespoons maple syrup

  10 soaked Deglet dates (soaked in ¼ cup warm water at least 1 hour. Reserve water). Dates may be soaked overnight. If using Medjool dates, fewer dates may be used.

  granola (Optional)

Put all ingredients, except granola, in a blender. Pulse to blend. You may have to scrape down the sides. Process on high until smooth. Serve immediately, topped with granola, if desired. Yields 4 servings. Store covered for 4 days.

Snacks

Nut Butters

Nut butters are very easy to make and don't take much time. They are so much healthier than buying them in the store because you know exactly what goes in them.

There are many nuts and seeds that make good nut butter. They include nuts like almonds, walnuts, cashews, pecans, and hazelnuts. Be sure to choose raw nuts, organic when possible.

3 cups raw nuts

Preheat oven to 350 degrees. Put raw nuts on a baking sheet and roast for 8 to 12 minutes, depending on the nuts you choose. Roast until the nuts are slightly golden brown. Let nuts cool. Add cooled roasted nuts to a food processor or blender and blend on medium speed until a creamy butter forms – up to 12 minutes or more. Scrape down the sides as needed. Once the butter is creamy, you can add a bit of healthy sea salt to taste, if you like. Store in a glass jar in the refrigerator for up to 3 or 4 weeks.

Notes: You can be creative with flavors and add pure vanilla extract, hemp or flaxseed or even chocolate.

Sweet Potato Chips and Fries

Coconut oil, for tossing
5 sweet potatoes peeled and slice. If making fries, cut into 1/4-inch long slices, then 1/4-wide inch strips. If you have a crinkle cut knife, use that. If making chips, slice thin on a mandolin.
Pink Himalayan sea salt
Cinnamon

Preheat oven to 400 degrees F. In a large bowl toss sweet potato with melted coconut oil to coat. Sprinkle with salt. Spread sweet potatoes in single layer on baking sheet, being sure not to overcrowd. Bake until sweet potatoes are tender and golden brown, turning occasionally, about 20 minutes. Sprinkle with cinnamon. Let cool 5 to 10 minutes before serving.

Breakfast

Gluten-free Muffins

1 cup organic gluten-free flour (I use Bob's Red Mill All-purpose Gluten-free Flour)

½ teaspoon baking soda

1 teaspoon aluminum-free baking powder

2 teaspoons cinnamon

1 tablespoon organic ground flaxseed

2 tablespoons organic gluten-free oats

1 ripe banana

½ cup finely chopped walnuts

1 egg

¼ cup melted coconut oil

2 tablespoons pure maple syrup

½ cup coconut or almond milk

In a small bowl, combine flour, baking soda, baking powder, cinnamon, flax, and oats. Stir to combine. In a medium bowl combine 1 egg, ¼ cup melted coconut oil, 2 tablespoons pure maple syrup, ½ cup coconut or almond milk. Mix well and add dry ingredients. Stir to combine. Mash the banana and stir banana and walnuts into to the batter. Let sit while oven heats to 375 degrees. Grease 6 muffin cups with coconut oil or organic vegetable shortening or line with paper muffin cups. Spoon batter into muffin cups. Bake for approx. 20 minutes or until a toothpick comes out clean.

Note: You may substitute 1 flax egg for the egg. To make a flax egg combine 1 tablespoon of ground flaxseed mixed with 2.5 tablespoons water – let sit for 5 minutes. Instead of the banana and walnuts, you may substitute 1 cup frozen mixed berries OR dried cranberries with a zest of lime OR 1 cup shredded carrots and 1/2 cup raisins.

Healthier Pancakes – Template Recipe

This recipe is a template recipe for healthier pancakes. You can switch it up by using banana, pumpkin or applesauce and change up the spices. It's a great base recipe you make many ways.

1 cup flour – garbanzo bean flour or gluten-free all-purpose flour or unbleached, unbromated wheat flour or ½ cup flour and 1/2 cup oat flour

2 teaspoons aluminum-free baking powder

1 tsp spices (cinnamon or ½ tsp cinnamon, ½ tsp nutmeg (optional)

1 tablespoon sweetener – (coconut sugar, maple sugar, honey, stevia)

½ cup of a binder – 1 egg or ½ cup pumpkin puree or flax egg substitute or 1 ripe mashed banana OR ½ cup applesauce.

1 tablespoon fat – coconut oil

1 cup liquid – coconut milk, almond milk, organic cow's milk

Mix dry ingredients together in a bowl. Combine binder, fat and liquid in a separate bowl. Pour wet ingredients into dry ingredients and whisk together until smooth. Preheat a griddle or electric skillet to medium-low heat and grease with coconut oil. Spoon about 1/3 cup of batter onto hot griddle. Cook until bubbles form on top and edges look dry. Flip pancake and cook another 2 to 3 minutes.

Shake Recipes

There are so many delicious combinations of shakes or smoothies that are only limited by your imagination. Here are just some of the things you can add to your healthy, plant-based protein.

Popular Combinations

Greens – Fresh baby spinach, basil, arugula, kale, mint

Fruits – ½ a green apple, ½ frozen banana, fresh or frozen strawberries, blueberries, raspberries, mango, peaches, kiwi, avocado

Essential Oils – add a drop or two of a food-grade essential oil like doTERRA brand – peppermint, grapefruit, wild orange, lemon, lime

Other (for added nutrition)– cacao, maca, ground flax seed, chia seeds, hemp seeds, chlorella, gluten-free oats

Strawberry/Banana Shake

8 oz water or almond, hemp or coconut milk

½ frozen banana

4 or 5 frozen strawberries

Vanilla or chocolate protein shake mix

(if using vanilla, add 2 tablespoons cacao powder)

A handful of ice cubes

Blend all together in a high-speed blender until smooth.

Green Apple/Avocado

8 oz water or almond, hemp or coconut milk

½ green apple, chopped

1 handful of baby spinach

½ avocado (pit and skin removed)

Vanilla protein shake mix

A handful of ice cubes

Blend all together in a high-speed blender until smooth.

Chocolate Almond Oat

8 oz water or almond, hemp or coconut milk

2 tablespoons gluten-free oats

1 – 2 tablespoons almond butter

Chocolate protein shake mix

A handful of ice cubes

Blend all together in a high-speed blender until smooth

Notes about ingredients

Spinach and kale will not add much--if any--flavor to your shake. Don't be afraid to add it for added nutrition. Arugula, however, will add a very interesting peppery flavor.

Cacao, as opposed to cocoa, not only adds delicious chocolate flavor, it also adds amazing nutrients to any shake. Cacao has 40 times the antioxidants as blueberries. It is also high in iron, magnesium, and calcium. It is a natural mood enhancer and anti-depressant.

Lunch or Dinner

Honey Lime Salad Dressing

Juice of 1 lime

1 tablespoon olive oil

2 teaspoons honey

¼ teaspoon paprika

¼ teaspoon turmeric

1/8 teaspoon black pepper

1/8 teaspoon sea salt

Mix all ingredients in a small bowl and whisk together. Pour over any salad. This recipe makes enough dressing for 1 or 2 individual salads.

Chili

1-pound ground (grass-fed) beef or venison or ground turkey

1 medium onion, diced

1 28oz can organic diced or crushed tomatoes

1 16 oz can organic tomato sauce

1 can kidney beans

2 tablespoons chili powder

1 tablespoon fresh minced garlic

½ teaspoon sea salt

½ teaspoon black pepper

½ teaspoon oregano

½ teaspoon cumin

½ teaspoon cayenne pepper

½ teaspoon paprika

Brown the meat in a skillet and drain, if necessary. Add onions and cook until onions are opaque. Add remaining ingredients and cook until heated through. Serve with avocado slices, if desired.

Chipotle Black Bean and Rice Skillet

> 1 tablespoon coconut oil
>
> ½ small onion
>
> 1 cup brown rice, cooked
>
> Juice from ½ lime
>
> ¼ cup water
>
> 2 teaspoons chipotle powder
>
> 1/3 cup black beans (drained and rinsed)
>
> 1-2 handfuls of fresh spinach
>
> ¼ cup cilantro (chopped)

In a skillet, heat coconut oil over medium heat. Add onion and cook until onion is opaque - about 5 -6 minutes. Add cooked rice, lime and chipotle powder, black beans, and water. Cook and stir until rice and beans are heated. Incorporate spinach and cilantro, stirring until spinach begins to wilt. If you'd like, you can make a hollow in the center of the skillet and crack one or two eggs into the center. Cover and let cook until egg whites are set, and yolk is done to desired firmness (7-12 minutes). Top with avocado or salsa, if desired. Serve immediately.

These are just a few of the recipes I use. I share many more in my 6-month coaching program and on my website.

CONCLUSION

I want to thank you for purchasing and reading this book. I want to encourage everyone to take charge of your health by eating mindfully. Pay attention to what you are putting in and on your body. Don't fall prey to the advertisers' ploys to get you to buy their products. The laws and guidelines governing products, including food products, are minimums to keep you from getting really sick. The issue is that over time, these toxins accumulate in the body and can do long-term damage.

Don't give in to your kids wanting those colorful sugary cereals, candy, pop and other sugary drinks, and toxic snacks and treats. Stand your ground, especially if your kids are young. They will thank you later.

The payoff is a life of health; feeling great, few, if any doctors' visits and medications, more energy, better sleep, fewer sick days. Think of the savings in the long run. Consider the cost of buying organic and eating healthy VS the cost of doctors, hospitals, medications and possibly a shorter time with your loved ones. You owe it to yourself and your families.

My mission is to change the face of health care in this country; to educate and coach people to better health the natural way through health coaching and public speaking.

I offer both private and group coaching. I use proven methods and natural products and I'm here to help in any way that I can.

I would love to get your feedback on this book. My prayer is that it has been a blessing to you in some way. Do me a huge favor and visit my website to leave me a comment.

<u>www.cleanfoodcleanyou.com</u>

If you would like a portable copy of the list of Toxins in Personal Care Products to carry with you when you shop, send me an email with this in the subject line (List of Toxins in Personal Care Products). I'll be happy to send that to you.

<u>Cleanfoodcleanyou@gmail.com</u>

ABOUT THE AUTHOR

Lisa Kafer has dedicated her life to helping others. She volunteers a few times a month as a speaker on the topic of plant-based eating and healthy living. She also teaches healthy cooking classes to children and adults, providing the essential building blocks for a more vibrant life. She's been instrumental in bettering the lives of her clients by coaching them in the areas of clean eating, detoxing and weight loss. She's written numerous published articles on various clean food topics as well as being featured on several news segments for local area television shows.

Lisa is a devoted wife and mother and resides in southwest Missouri amidst a happy farm full of animals. She's passionate about educating, empowering and inspiring people to live their best, healthiest life possible well into old age. She values her small-town community and enjoys working with local family-owned farms and businesses. She's active in a wide network of healers and helpers and is ever pursuant of information to share. Helping people is at the root of everything she does, and it's because of this passion that she's expanded her business, written her first book, and taken to the internet to spread the word about clean eating, hoping to inspire better living to a broader range of people. In her spare time (when that occasionally happens), she enjoys riding horses, photography, and relaxed family time.

Cleanfoodcleanyou@gmail.com
www.cleanfoodcleanyou.com
www.facebook.com/417cleanfoodcleanyou